Coconut Oil

The Ultimate Guide To Using Coconut Oil for Weight Loss, Allergies, and Longevity

KARA AIMER

CONTENTS

INTRODUCTION

What comes to mind when someone mentions coconut oil? Do you think of it as the oil that you use for cooking? Or do you think of it as the oil you apply on your skin or hair? Well, if you are the type that thinks that all fats make you fat, then you are probably on the camp that stands for the idea that coconut oil makes you fat (after all, it is a fat!).

Whatever it is you think about coconut oil, I can bet that you probably don't use the oil in as many aspects of your life as you should. Do you know that you can use it for fighting allergies, dealing with different skin problems, fighting hair loss, losing weight and in many other ways? If you didn't know, now you do.

If you are wondering what is in coconut oil that makes it so good for all the different uses, this book is just perfect for you. It will introduce you to the world of using coconut oil so that you can discover the endless possibilities of using coconut oil. You will be amazed at all the things you can use coconut oil for that you had no idea you could use.

SIMPLE FACTS ABOUT COCONUT OIL

It is essential that we understand some important facts about coconut oil before we can look at how you can use this super fat. Coconut oil can be described as edible oil that is extracted from meat or kernel of mature coconut kernel. It's made up of about 90 percent of saturated fats, 3 percent of poly-unsaturated fats and 6 percent of mono-unsaturated fats. As opposed to other highly unsaturated or saturated fats, this oil is composed of medium-chain fatty acids commonly abbreviated as MCFAs. The presence of saturated fat in coconut gives it the heat-stable properties along with a long shelf life.

This oil is one of the super-foods that is unique in terms of health benefits and uses, as it is a good remedy for weight loss, skin and hair care, for curing allergies and for general longevity. This has made coconut oil to be widely used in traditional medicines and as a carrier oil in pharmaceutical firms. Here are some facts about coconut oil that are worth noting:

1. Coconut oil is a rich source of energy, as only 100 grams yields around 884 calories. This means that a single gram of coconut oil has 9 calories, and thus may not be recommended if on a calorie-restricted diet. But with moderation, you can enjoy the many benefits the oil possesses.

2. This oil is rich in saturated fats and thus is a stable vegetable cooking oil with a long shelf life. Due to its high smoke point of 450 degrees F, it's majorly used for deep-frying.

3. Since it is a saturated fatty acid, coconut oil is a medium-chain fatty acid that is composed of 6 to 12 atoms of carbons. The medium chain triglycerides that are present in coconut oil include lauric acid, caproic acid,

capric acid and caprylic acid. The fatty acids amount to 68 percent saturated and 59 percent of the total fat content.

4. Lauric acid, a carbon-12 saturated fat, contributes the highest portion of the fatty acids, being about 25 percent of the total content of fat.

5. The medium chains triglycerides in coconut oil are directly absorbed into the blood stream, which bring an early sense of satiety. The MCTs are also useful in raising the concentration of good cholesterol levels or HDL in the blood.

6. Cold-pressed coconut oil has a little amount of vitamin E plus other tocopherols with 100 grams of the oil containing about 0.2mcg of vitamin E.

7. You don't have to keep coconut oil under refrigeration; just store into a bottle in the kitchen cupboard or any safe place. The oil is solid at temperatures below 76 Fahrenheit and liquefies at temperatures above that.

It is important to understand that there are different types of coconut oil. So, what are these types of coconut oil and how are they used?

TYPES OF COCONUT OIL

Generally, there are two types of coconut oil; the one produced from fresh coconut and requires no or less refining and the coconut oil from mass production at an industrial level. Coconut oil is available as a naturally refined product as the oil has to be extracted from the whole coconut. The unrefined coconut oil is the oil still inside the coconut meat from the coconut off a tree. The little-refined oil is often referred to as 'virgin' coconut oil, a term used to show the natural nature of coconut oil.

Refined Coconut Oil

This variety of coconut oil is extracted from dried coconut that is also known as copra (copra is a term used to describe coconut oil that comes from dried coconut shell but is inedible thus requiring refining). The copra can be produced in a variety of ways among them kiln drying, sun drying, smoke drying or a combination of the methods. This oil is also referred to as refined, bleached and deodorized oil or RBD oil. This oil has to undergo processing as the dried copra is not proper for consumption but has to undergo the refining process. The processing helps to remove impurities and stabilizes coconut oil, especially because it is mass-produced.

The refined variety of coconut oil is usually odorless and tasteless, and can withstand higher cooking temperatures. Since the oil reaches the smoke point after a longer time, it is excellent for deep-frying of food with pure and malleable fat without the coconut flavor left behind. However, this variety does not offer the required benefits of the completely raw and unrefined coconut oil. The sad point is that the majority of coconut oil sold at your grocery or other food stores is the refined coconut oil, unless stated as otherwise.

That said, the refined coconut oil still has the same medium chain fatty acids and is close to virgin coconut oil based on nutritional values. Furthermore, not all refined oils are similar; look for the un-hydrogenated variety that is refined from natural and chemical free process such as steam distillation. If on a budget, you may still consider the cheaper refined coconut for deep-frying, in soaps and bath oils or as a body moisturizer. There are various categories of refined coconut oil:

Expeller-pressed Coconut Oils

This type is mainly used for mass production in tropical countries through physical or mechanical refining from copra. This type of refining is cleaner compared to chemical refining that uses solvent extracts among them 'hexane'.

Coconut oil

In most cases, a product with this term is used to refer to the RBD coconut oil coming from copra and refined into non-edible uses. This type of coconut oil is used to make detergents and cleaning products though some companies are manufacturing edible coconut oil products. The cheaper oils are produced from mass production using solvent extraction (there are concerns whether those solvents still remain in coconut). The recommendable option is to purchase coconut oil not refined through solvents.

Liquid Coconut Oil

This is a form of edible coconut oil that is promoted as being able to remain liquid even under refrigeration. The variety also known as MCT oil is made from fractional distillation and has the Lauric acid removed. The liquid coconut oil is mostly used in making skin care products, as well as dietary supplements. Since Lauric acid is a saturated fatty acid, when it is removed from liquid coconut oil, it leaves a product with a lower melting point. Due to this, this kind of coconut oil is a highly refined coconut oil without the most important component of coconut oil.

Unrefined Coconut Oil

This variety of coconut oil is extracted from fresh coconut as opposed from copra though it's not a standard term for all unrefined oils. Unrefined oil is normally labeled as 'virgin' or 'extra-virgin', meaning that it's made from raw coconut oil through a mechanical process. Based on the process of extraction, it can have mild to intense flavor, as longer exposures to heat results into more flavored oil. When buying virgin coconut oil, find out whether it is produced from copra or coconut. Where a copra-base is used, then this is not true virgin oil. The unrefined raw virgin coconut oil ought to have a mild coconut flavor and scent. There isn't such difference between extra virgin and virgin coconut oil, thus 'extra virgin' labeling would be a trick to make you pay more. A number of industries may even put a 'virgin coconut' label for standard RBD as a marketing strategy. The virgin or unrefined oil is more beneficial and superior to the refined oil.

Based on the virgin oils sold in food stores, the unrefined coconut oil falls into two groups based on the production methods:

By pressing dried coconut

This virgin oil variety is made from pressing oil out of a dried coconut, where fresh coconut meat is dried and later the oil is pressed out. This extraction method is preferred for the mass production of virgin coconut oil. Desiccated or dried coconut is well established and is preferred by most industries to make virgin coconut products. It's the most common virgin or 'extra virgin' in stores today and it has a higher nutritional and medicinal value than the RBD coconut oil.

From wet milling process

The virgin oil from this process is extracted from fresh coconut meat without having to dry it first. Coconut meat is pressed to release coconut milk where coconut oil is separated from the water. To separate the coconut oil from coconut water, methods such as refrigeration, fermentation, boiling, enzymes, and mechanical centrifuge are applicable. Coconut oil made from fermentation process has the highest quality, as it uses heat. Use of heat in extraction yields highest amounts of antioxidants in the oil.

A fermentation process is a simple process you can even practice in your kitchen. You start by preparing coconut milk emulsion from freshly grated coconut, and then allow the milk to sit and ferment overnight. The water is heavier than oil so it sinks to the bottom of your bowl, and a clear layer of coconut is left on top. To get the virgin oil, you only have to scope it out using any reliable method and out into a big container. You then heat the coconut oil constantly until you get coconut solids falling to the bottom of your pan. Finally, filter to get coconut oil.

Buying Coconut Oil

Since different coconut oil manufacturers use different techniques in production and marketing, you may have to try out various brands to determine the best. Expensive coconut oil brands do not always mean that the coconut oil is pure since most products do not show the quality of ingredients used and the level of purity. The factors below will be of great help in helping you buy the best kind of coconut oil:

Aroma and flavor: Raw virgin and unrefined oil have a mild coconut taste and smell. Coconut oil tasting or smelling like something roasted or smoky may mean that it is over-exposed to heat, which means that it has probably lost much of its nutrients. In case the coconut oil seems to be neutral in taste and odorless, it must be treated or refined.

Color: Pure coconut oil should be white in color when in solid form, or colorless in liquid form. Any alterations or discoloring means that the coconut has been contaminated and it's inferior.

The next chapters will address the various ways that you can use coconut oil and enjoy its amazing benefits.

COCONUT OIL FOR FOOD PREPARATION AND HOME REMEDIES

Some of the amazing ways of using coconut oil include in cooking, for cold treatment, to cure bruises and cuts and other skin care routine applications. For edible coconut oil, try consuming 3-4 tablespoons of coconut oil as an adult per day and a little fewer amounts for kids. In case, it's your first time experimenting with saturated fat or if under low-fat diet, start gradually and then gradually increase your consumption. This may prevent possible problems such as initial diarrhea.

Coconut Oil In Food Preparation
The most applicable use of coconut oil at your home is food preparation, where you can use it in the following ways:

*Coconut oil is very heat stable thus a good product for cooking, where you can use it for deep-frying. You can also use it on stir-fries, sauces, roast meats etc.

*Coconut oil is a good butter or margarine since it is usually solid most times of the day even when out of the fridge. You can use coconut oil when preparing desserts, baked goods, spreads, and dips. The recommended amount is a 1:1 ratio when using in place of other oils, to make, for instance, pan-fried meatballs, cherry ripe chocolate truffles, or grain-free granola.

*You can use the best raw unrefined virgin coconut oil to make mayonnaise, or add few teaspoons of the oil to coffee, tea, juices, and smoothies.

*You may combine a little coconut oil with honey and cacao to create an efficient energy booster before you do a workout.

Coconut Oil For Home Remedies

In addition to being used in food, you can use coconut oil in your home for various remedies such as:

1. You can use it to treat and fully eliminate head lice

2. You can use coconut oil to kill yeast, yeast infections, toe fungus and athletes foot. This is possible due to coconut oil's antifungal properties.

3. You can create a homemade vapor rub by combining a few drops of rosemary and eucalyptus oils with a ½ cup of coconut oil. Then use this mixture to rub on your chest and throat.

4. To treat skin problems on pets such bruises, just apply a little amount of the oil on them.

COCONUT OIL FOR WEIGHT LOSS

Coconut oil is used for weight loss due to the following properties:

It controls weight

A scientific study conducted in 2009 to find out the connection between coconut oil and weight loss in women concluded that it reduces obesity. This is because coconut oil is quickly digested and absorbed into the blood thus providing instant energy, which reduces the need to overeat. Additionally, it controls insulin resistance, which if not controlled can lead to obesity and diabetes. To use coconut oil for weight loss, just add about a teaspoon of the oil to food. You can then continually increase the consumption to 4 teaspoons daily.

Coconut oil boosts metabolism

Consumption of about 2 tablespoons of coconut oil daily has been found to burn a high number of kilojoules of fat. For now, obesity tends to be the biggest health problem that is caused by not only the consumption of high-calorie foods but also the sources of calories play a significant role. Actually, different foods will affect your body and hormonal activity in a distinct way, thus calories are very different.

Though coconut oil contains a high level of calories, the MCFAs found in the oil can raise the amount of energy that the body spends compared to other long-chain fats. Consuming 15-30 grams of MCTs daily raises the daily energy expenditure by around 5 percent. Therefore, taking about 120 calories of coconut oil can burn more fat by raising your energy expenditure. The effectiveness of metabolic system assists your body to keep the weight off and boost the immune system.

Stops sugar cravings

To minimize the temptation to snack on sugar and highly processed foods, try consuming a teaspoon of virgin coconut oil to stop the sugar cravings. Eating of more fats brings more satiety than consumption of carbs, which means that you will feel lesser cravings. As such, this will help you to cut down on sugar. Additionally, constant hunger is one of the reasons that can easily lead to overeating. However, consuming coconut can make you feel full hence no need to consume more food.

Coconut oil makes you eat less

In addition to reducing sugar cravings, coconut oil reduces your hunger and thus makes you eat less without even trying. On average, taking of 2 teaspoons of coconut oil can reduce your daily calorie intake by 256. A different health study found out that eating more MCTs at breakfast could significantly lower the calories you consume during lunch.

Coconut oil can burn stubborn abdominal fat

Coconut oil has been shown to lower the stubborn fat around the abdomen and other body organs. Abdominal fat is the most dangerous type of fat as it results to many health problems. The circumference of your waist is an indication of the amount of fats in the abdominal cavity.

An ounce or 30 ml of coconut oil daily has shown a good effect on reduction of waist circumference and the BMI within 3 months. In men, consumption of an ounce of coconut oil can reduce your weight circumference by 1.1 inches within a month. When you add other weight burning strategies such as eating less calories and exercising, you will definitely experience a change in your waist circumference.

COCONUT OIL FOR HEALTHY SKIN AND HAIR

Coconut oil is the best face moisturizer, great for skin and provides amazing nourishment to your hair. Actually, coconut oil cannot compare with artificial skin and hair care products that contain a lot of water. This water meant to offer the moisturizing properties soon dries and leaves the skin very dry and to some extent dehydrated. Furthermore, a number of commercial products have petrol-based ingredients, which can suffocate your skin.

Coconut oil offers the deepest and real moisturizing properties. It assists in giving strength to the underlying tissues as it also removes the dead cells stuck on the surface of the skin. The oil is also good for providing some shin to your hair. To get these rare benefits, just rub a small amount of coconut oil on the dry ends of your hair to restore that shine and glory. For face use, apply coconut oil as an ordinary moisturizer.

Coconut oil at first appears to be of grease consistency but soon after application, it is absorbed into the skin leaving it looking dry and smooth. You only need just a spoonful to moisturize your entire body, while using it as your regular lotion. The following are some of the other benefits of coconut oil:

Slows fine line formation on the face
Coconut oil is an effective moisturizing agent for the skin and it helps maintain the connective tissues firm, and combat sagging and wrinkles. To obtain this benefit, just apply the oil directly on the skin to soften the appearance on the fine lines. Alternatively, you can use coconut oil for your body and face. The best variety of coconut oil to use is the virgin coconut that has no additives or flavors.

Lauric acid kills microorganisms

Lauric acid is almost 50 percent of the total fatty acids in coconut oil, which when digested through enzymes is converted to monolaurin, a form of a monoglyceride. Both monolaurin and Lauric acid are effective in killing fungi, viruses and bacteria. Coconut oil is strong against pathogens such as Staphylococcus Aureus bacteria and Candida Albicans, a common yeast fungus that causes human infections.

Coconut oil is also applicable on other protection cases such as killing harmful bacteria in the mouth through oil pulling; this mouthwash can boost your dental health and effectively combat bad breath.

Protects against skin and hair damage

Coconut oil is useful for cosmetic purposes to boost the general health and appearance of the skin and hair. In fact, research has proven that coconut oil can improve the moisture and lipid content in a person suffering from dry skin. The oil is also effective in preventing damage of hair and is a great sunscreen. As a sunscreen, it inhibits about 20 percent of UV rays from affecting the skin.

Used as a massage oil

Coconut oil is good for smooth and healthy skin and thus is used for massages. The oil is solid at room temperature, which means that it is less messy compared to other liquid oils when used for body massage. Massaging with coconut oil relaxes and moisturizes the skin. To massage the skin, just add 4-5 tablespoons of coconut oil to a hot tub and then gently bath or massage in the oil for soft and hydrated skin.

Used to make homemade products

You can use coconut oil to make natural homemade products among them deodorants, bug repellants, toothpaste, and homemade soaps. All you need to do, for instance, when making soap, is to use it as a base and the coconut oil assist will assist in hardening the soap as well as breaking down other oils and grease. Just add a little amount of it when making soap. When making soap, you only need a few ingredients, which include lye, water, and coconut oil. The good thing about coconut oil is that it is organic and does not have side effects posed by other commercial products.

As a hair conditioner

Sometimes your outer hair shaft can become rumpled and out of shape, which means that you require a remedy to put everything back into place. Coconut oil can be used both on your hair ends as well as on the entire scalp or head for deep conditioning. To use coconut oil as an overnight conditioner for your hair, just rub a little amount of oil into the hair ends then comb through your hair and keep the hair in a loose bun before going to bed. Wash the hair the following morning.

Used as a static reducer

Use coconut oil on the hair as a static reducer by rubbing your hands together using a little amount of coconut oil on them. Later, run your hair through the static hair.

As a moisturizer

Coconut oil has great moisturizing and healing properties that allow it to be used as regular lotion. When used effectively, the oil easily penetrates the skin to deliver a refreshing and smooth feeling. Ignore the greasy appearance coconut oil has since as soon as it dries, it leaves you with hydrated skin. After applying onto your skin, allow a few minutes for it to dry and restore the skin tone.

Similarly, use it on the hair by rubbing a little amount, wrap with a towel overnight and later shampoo as usual. After doing the dishes, your hands may become dry and scaly thus you should apply coconut oil on your hands after washing.

Used as an exfoliating body scrub

Use coconut oil as a base for face or body scrubs, by just melting it, stirring in sugar and allowing to cool before using. Alternatively, you can melt ½ cup coconut oil and transfer it to a tin, then add 2-4 tablespoons of brown or white sugar. Allow it to cool or keep in the fridge to solidify and then remove from the tin or mold. To use as a scrub, just slice off a little piece and scrub on your damp face or body gently; rinse off and later apply your favorite moisturizer.

As a make-up remover

It is essential to remove makeup at the end of the day if you want to have healthy skin. Therefore, you can use coconut oil to remove makeup and restore your natural skin tone. Scoop a little amount of coconut oil and then quickly rub it over your face in a circular motion to eliminate any traces of the make-up and later pat dry the skin. Coconut oil is effective on all types of eye make-ups whether waterproof or not. Once done with coconut oil, you can wash with soap and rinse.

As a diaper cream

Coconut oil has antifungal and antibacterial properties that allow it to be used to moisturize the body. Due to this property, coconut oil is a great choice for baby salve or all natural diaper cream, which is also safe to use with cloth diapers. Just melt coconut oil with a little Shea butter and whip the 2 until it turns solid. Then apply the mixture as required to the affected areas to heal irritation.

As a sunscreen

Coconut oil is an effective treatment against skin burns, skin cellulite and as an after-shave lotion.

BOOST YOUR IMMUNE SYSTEM AND DIGESTION WITH COCONUT OIL

Coconut oil eases digestion

In case you are dealing with poor digestion or possible bloating, coconut oil can help a lot to improve digestion. The oil is effective in curing digestive disorders among them irritable bowel syndrome and tummy bugs caused by pathogens. The fatty acids in coconut oil have antimicrobial properties that sooth your digestive system thus relieving poor digestion.

Coconut oil improves your immunity

Coconut oil is made of capric acid, caprylic acid, and Lauric acid, each of which has antimicrobial properties that improve the immune system. Lauric acid has the highest quantity of fatty acids, 75 percent of which is converted into monolaurin. This conversion is effective in healing Candida, helicobacter pylori, cytomegalovirus, influenza and herpes to boost immunity.

Coconut oil can boost brain function

The fatty acid present in coconut oil can heal Alzheimer's symptoms, a condition that results into dementia. This disease is mostly persistent in elderly persons, as they seem to have lower ability to metabolize glucose for energy in various brain organs. Fatty acids are metabolized into ketone bodies that instead supply energy to the brain. Ketones have been quoted by multiple health experts as being able to heal malfunctioning cells and curing Alzheimer's disease. Numerous studies have found that coconut oil can instantly improve brain functioning especially in victims with mild form of Alzheimer's disease.

Relieves constipation

To improve your digestion and relief constipation, just take a tablespoon of coconut oil each breakfast especially on an empty stomach. This helps keep the digestive system working effectively. For better results, try using 2 tablespoons of coconut oil to address constipation problems.

Has healing properties

Diseases such as common colds and flu, ulcers, urinary tract infections, pneumonia, and cavities weaken the immune system. Coconut oil is effective in treating the bacteria and influenza viruses responsible for these conditions. Coconut oil also eliminates fungal infections like yeast and excess Candida, which may weaken your immune system seriously and even lower the pH of your blood. You can add coconut oil to your diet to keep your immune system strong throughout the seasons especially in winter.

Coconut oil is good for oral health

Since coconut oil is effective in killing bacteria living in the mouth, research has found out a link between oral health and overall health. Actually, poor oral health can release more bacteria to your entire system and actually harm the internal organs. Coconut oil can effectively reduce the number of dangerous bacteria living in the mouth and thus boost your overall health as well.

Coconut oil as a digestive aid

Apart from healing constipation, coconut oil is a digestive aid in terms of treating acid indigestion and acid reflux. In addition to treating these common symptoms, the oil can treat other serious stomach problems such as Cohn's disease and ulcerative colitis. This is because the oil has anti-microbial properties that fight inflammation and other infections. This makes it a great remedy for gut and intestinal-related problems.

COCONUT OIL FOR TREATING ALLERGIES AND FOR OPTIMAL HEALTH

Treats allergies

Though there may be other methods of eliminating specific allergies such as hay fever, coconut oil is effective in treating chronic or seasonal allergies. Additionally, coconut oil is a great remedy for combating allergies resulting from certain foods like dairy, peanuts, gluten, wheat, and soy. Ensure that you are not allergic to coconut oil before you use it to treat allergies.

Addresses seizures

Coconut oil is effective in minimizing occurrence of seizures, as the fatty acids from coconut oil are easily converted into ketones. Actually, coconut oil forms part of the ketogenic diet, characterized by high intake of fat but low carbohydrates. This diet has been found to treat a number of disorders such as the drug-resistant epilepsy in children.

Deals with insulin resistance

A scientific study found out that coconut oil is effective in preventing insulin resistance, thus controlling the risk of developing type 2 Diabetes. The medium chain fatty acids are easily absorbed into the cells and are quickly converted to energy. This overall process improves the sensitivity to insulin.

Prevents loss of bones

A metabolic disorder associated with oxidative stress and free radicals leads to the development of osteoporosis and bone loss. Taking extra-virgin coconut oil can effectively maintain the structure of your bones and reduce weakening of bones or osteoporosis. Coconut oil has sufficient amounts of polyphenols and antioxidants, and you only need to consume up to 3 tablespoons for good results.

Fights cancer

Due to the medium-chain triglycerides found in coconut oil, the oil has shown ability to offer an antitumor effect and maintain a healthy immune system. Though coconut oil may not cure all types of cancer, research has shown its potential.

Fights Inflammation

Inflammation of the kidneys and liver can be very risky for overall health. This is because inflammations actually lead to many chronic diseases such as arthritis. Taking of few tablespoons of virgin coconut oil that is prepared without high-heat or chemical involvement can help treat chronic inflammation.

Balancing of hormones

Coconut oil contains plenty of healthy fats that facilitate healthy adrenal and thyroid glands, which can help in lowering the level of cortisol (stress hormone) to balance the hormones. Coconut oil is also great in addressing inflammation along with maintaining a healthy metabolism; two factors that affect balancing of hormones. Coconut oil also has Lauric acid, a compound that supports a healthy adrenal and thyroid. Likewise, this helps control stress hormone, cortisol, thus balancing your hormones.

As a sleep aid

Lack of sleep is mostly brought by problems such as stress and anxiety. Coconut oil is a great carrier oil when making a soothing and relaxing essential oils remedy at home. Just combine roman chamomile oil or lavender essential oils with a little amount of coconut and apply it on your temples to relax and sleep well.

CONCLUSION

It is quite amazing that one simple oil can do so much. The only way that you can enjoy the amazing benefits of coconut oil is to start using it. A point of caution when it comes to ingesting coconut oil for weight loss is that you need to reduce your calorie intake so that intake of coconut oil can balance that calorie difference. Simply eating the same amount of calories and adding coconut oil can actually lead to weight gain rather than weight loss, so watch out on that.

Good luck, and congratulations on starting your path toward a happier, healthier, and more wholesome you!

Finally, if you enjoyed this book, please share your thoughts and post a positive review on Amazon. I would greatly appreciate your support!

Thank you and good luck!

Kara Aimer

ADDITIONAL RESOURCES

Please point your web browser to **www.plaid-enterprises.com** for more related resources, my full bibliography and to grab your FREE book!

www.ingramcontent.com/pod-product-compliance
Lightning Source LLC
Chambersburg PA
CBHW070942290526
45795CB00003B/1114